Respiratory System Nursing Test Review

Master Nursing School and the NCLEX Exam 110
Practice Test Questions with Rationales

Nursestudy.Net

Contents

How This Book Is Set Up

All 110 questions are in the front part of
this book. The questions are repeated
with the answers and rationale immediately following the questions in the
second half of this book. This allows
the reader to take the test and check answers in the back of the
book or skip
to the back and review questions and answers at the same time.

Introduction

I want to thank you and congratulate you for downloading the book, *"Respiratory System Nursing Test Review."*

By

Anna Curran, RN, BSN, PHN

Emergency Room Registered Nurse

Critical Care Transport Nurse

Clinical Nurse Instructor for LVN and BSN students

Anna began writing materials to help her BSN and LVN students with their studies. She takes the topics that the students are learning and expands on them to try to help with their understanding of the nursing process. Her experience spans over two decades in nursing, starting as an LVN in 1993. She received her RN license in 1997. She has worked in Medical-Surgical, Telemetry, ICU and the ER. She found a passion in the ER and has stayed in this department for 16 years. She is a clinical instructor for LVN and BSN students, along with a critical care transport nurse.

Thanks again for downloading this book. If you like the book, please leave us feedback and let us know.

Join me on

NurseStudy.Net

Facebook

Instagram

Careplans and More

Visit NurseStudy.net for over 1000 FREE Nursing Diagnosis and Nursing Careplans.

Get my FREE book on:
Pass The NCLEX RN & NCLEX PN: Test Taking Tips and Strategies to Easily Pass the NCLEX | Simple Fast and Easy Steps | Nursing Questions with Answers and Rationales

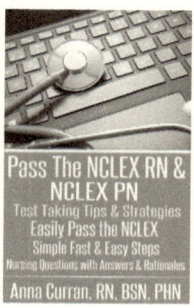

Get the FREE Book

Disclaimer

Every effort has been made to ensure that the information in this guide is correct. The publisher and author do not assume and hereby disclaim any liability to any party for any loss, disruption, or damage caused by errors and omissions, whether such errors or omissions result from accident, negligence, or any other cause.

This book is not intended as a substitute for the medical advice of physicians. The reader should regularly consult with a physician in matters relation to his or her health and particularly with respect to any signs and symptoms that may require diagnosis or medical attention.

the publisher, except in the case of brief quotations in embodied in the critical reviews and certain other noncommercial uses permitted by copyright law.

Respiratory Nursing Review Questions Without Answers or Rationales:

1. The first and most common symptom of emphysema is:

   a. Purulent sputum

   b. Episodic wheezing

   c. Cough

   d. Dyspnea

2. The physician suspects bronchiectasis in a patient. Which test will he ask the nurse to perform to confirm the diagnosis?

   a. Lung biopsy

   b. Chest CT scan

   c. Blood test

   d. Bronchoscopy

3. The "pink puffers" are the patients of disease:

a. Tuberculosis

b. Emphysema

c. Asthma

d. Pneumonia

4. A patient comes to the physician and complains of symptoms like shortness of breath, wheezing, and tightness in the chest for a few months. What could be the diagnosis of his condition?

a. Pneumothorax

b. Tuberculosis

c. Asthma

d. Pneumonia

5. A person suffering from asthma wants to get his wisdom tooth extracted. The dentist advised him to get a medical consent from his pulmonologist. What time will the pulmonologist advise him as the safest for getting the extraction done? (Select all that apply)

a. 9 AM

b. 11 AM

c. 2 PM

d. It is not safe at any time

6. A person comes to the clinic and gives a history of his wife complaining about snoring and gasping sounds while sleeping. He also complains of sudden awakenings sometimes at night. Which of these is a probable cause of these symptoms?

a. Apnea

b. Tuberculosis

c. Sleep apnea

d. Cold

7. Which of the following is an obstructive pulmonary disease? (Select all that apply)

a. Chronic bronchitis

b. Pneumonia

c. Asthma

d. Emphysema

8. Using systemic corticosteroid in the treatment of severe asthma can lead to (Select all that apply)

a. Alteration of fat distribution

b. Glucose intolerance

c. Excitation of CNS

d. Delayed wound healing

e. Churg-Strauss syndrome

9. According to the modified MRC dyspnea scale, breathlessness after walking for a few minutes on level ground is considered as a grade:

a. 1

b. 2

c. 3

d. 4

10. Select the key features of COPD. (Select all that apply)

a. Central cyanosis

b. Hyperinflated "barrel" chest

c. Non-palpable cardiac apex

d. Prolonged expiration

e. Use of accessory respiratory muscles

11. Select the incorrect statement.

a. The functional residual cavity is residual volume + Expiratory reserve volume

b. Total lung capacity is inspiratory reserve volume + tidal volume + expiratory reserve volume

c. Inspiratory capacity is inspiratory reserve volume + tidal volume

d. Vital capacity is tidal volume + inspiratory reserve volume + expiratory reserve volume

12. The bronchus is not the primary obstructed site in:

a. Asthma

b. Emphysema

c. Chronic bronchitis

d. Bronchiectasis

13. An asthmatic patient informs the nurse that he is feeling gastric disturbances a few days after he started his treatment. Which of the following drug is most likely present in his regimen?

a. Beclomethasone

b. Ipratropium

c. Theophylline

d. Montelukast

14. Which of the following drugs are contraindicated in an asthmatic patient? (Select all that apply)

a. Ibuprofen

b. Losartan

c. Aspirin

d. Propranolol

15. A genetic respiratory disease caused by the mutation of a gene on chromosome 7 is:

a. Primary ciliary dyskinesia

b. Cystic fibrosis

c. Tracheoesophageal fistula

d. None of the above

16. A baby born prematurely during the 28th week of embryonic growth. Which of the following respiratory structure is most likely to be least developed?

a. Trachea

b. Bronchioles

c. Lungs

d. Alveoli

17. A characteristic finding in the alveolus injured due to acute respiratory distress syndrome is:

a. Edema

b. Sloughed bronchial epithelium

c. Neutrophil sequestration and migration into alveolus

d. Hyaline membrane

18. While doing the lung examination, the nurse hears a fremitus sound. What can be the diagnosis based on this result?

a. Pneumothorax

b. Pleural effusion

c. Lobar pneumonia

d. Atelectasis

19. A hypertensive patient came to the physician with a complaint of dry cough for 3 weeks. Which of these sentences are correct for this patient? (Select all that apply)

a. The patient is taking furosemide for hypertension.

b. The drug prescribed for hypertension needs to be replaced by alternative drug

c. The patient should be prescribed dextromethorphan for treating the dry cough permanently.

d. The patient is under captopril medication for hypertension.

20. Pursed breathing is seen in: (Select all that apply)

a. Asthma

b. Chronic bronchitis

c. Emphysema

d. Bronchiectasis

21. Cervical or mediastinal lymphadenitis is commonly seen in:

a. Pulmonary tuberculosis

b. Miliary tuberculosis

c. Extrapulmonary tuberculosis

d. All the above

22. Clubbing of fingers is not seen due to:

a. Bronchiectasis

b. Lung abscess

c. Suppurative pneumonia

d. Massive pneumothorax

23. A nurse was assessing the chest wall movements in a patient. She observed bilateral diminished chest wall movements. What can be the diagnosis based on this finding?

a. Acute bronchitis

b. Bronchial asthma

c. Lobar collapse

d. Emphysema

24. A type of asthma in which the patient does not get free from symptoms in between subsequent asthmatic attacks is:

a. Atopic asthma

b. Status asthmaticus

c. Chronic asthma

d. non-atopic asthma

25. Which of the following is most commonly caused by aspiration of oropharyngeal contents?

a. Lung abscess

b. Lung cancer

c. Pneumonia

d. Pneumothorax

26. A patient is prescribed theophylline. What should the common adverse effect be informed to the patient?

a. Diarrhea

b. Tremors

c. Tachycardia

d. Candidiasis

27. Which of the following is caused by rhinovirus?

a. Nasal polyp

b. Rhinitis

c. Bronchitis

d. Nasopharyngeal carcinoma

28. Consolidation of an entire lobe of the lung visible in the chest X-ray of is a diagnostic feature of:

a. Lobar pneumonia

b. Bronchopneumonia

c. Aspiration pneumonia

d. Atypical pneumonia

29. A patient comes with a complaint of fever, cough, and difficulty in breathing for 8 days. He gives the history of alcohol consumption to the nurse. Which of the following can be the diagnosis based on this information?

a. Lobar pneumonia

b. Bronchopneumonia

c. Aspiration pneumonia

d. Atypical pneumonia

30. Which of the following is not prescribed to treat a dry cough?

a. Dextromethorphan

b. Codeine

c. Bromhexine

d. Noscapine

31. Which of these is not true for broncho-pneumonia?

a. Bronchial and bronchiolar inflammation is seen.

b. Consolidation is seen in an entire lobe.

c. More commonly seen in lower lobes.

d. None of these

32. A patient was recently admitted to the hospital with the symptoms of shortness of breath, fever, and cough. After looking at his chest X-ray, pneumonia was diagnosed. The patient gave the history of international travel 1 month ago. Which of these can be the most probable diagnosis? (Select all that apply)

a. Acute respiratory distress syndrome

b. Coronavirus disease

c. Severe acute respiratory syndrome

d. Tuberculosis

33. An organism that causes pneumonia and is the third most common cause of urinary tract infection is:

a. Streptococcus pneumonia

b. Klebsiella pneumonia

c. Legionella

d. Burkholderia pseudomallei

34. The physician asks the nurse to perform the methacholine test. Which of the following diagnosis does the physician want to confirm?

a. Asthma

b. Pneumonia

c. Chronic bronchitis

d. Tuberculosis

35. Microabsecess formation is a characteristic histologic feature of:

a. Community-acquired pneumonia

b. Suppurative pneumonia

c. Tuberculosis

d. Lobar pneumonia

36. "Ghon focus" is a diagnostic feature of:

a. Pneumonia

b. Chronic bronchitis

c. Emphysema

d. Tuberculosis

37. A pregnant woman is diabetic. Which of these respiratory diseases may occur in the baby?

a. Respiratory distress syndrome

b. Pneumonia

c. Acute bronchitis

d. Asthma

38. Increased hemoglobin concentration is seen in:

a. Anemia

b. Polycythemia

c. Leukemia

d. CO poisoning

39. Trauma in the region of Kiesselbach plexus can lead to:

a. Rhinosinusitis

b. Epistaxis

c. Deep vein thrombosis

d. Embolism

40. Which of the following drug can be added to the regimen if bronchodilator does not provide relief from asthma?

a. Inhaled steroid

b. High dose of steroid

c. Corticosteroid and a sequential therapeutic drug

d. Oral steroid

41. Lung abscess can be caused due to: (Select all that apply)

a. Pyogenic organisms

b. Thromboembolism of lung

c. M. tuberculosis

d. Smoking

42. Which of the following is not a cause of pleural effusion?

a. Increased production of the fluid

b. Reduced fluid absorption by pleura

c. Decreased capillary permeability

d. Increased hydrostatic pressure.

43. Which fluid is accumulated in chylothorax?

a. Blood

b. Pus

c. Chyme

d. Chyle

44. Select the incorrect statements for tuberculous pleural effusion. (Select all that apply)

a. Transudate fluid

b. Lymphocytes are predominant cells

c. The fluid is straw-colored

d. The fluid is blood-stained

45. The pathologic report of bronchi states the presence of Charcot-Leyden crystals. What can be the diagnosis based on this finding?

a. Emphysema

b. Chronic bronchitis

c. Asthma

d. Pneumonia

46. In the chest X-ray of a patient suffering from emphysema: (Select all that apply)

a. Anteroposterior diameter of the chest is increased

b. Diaphragm looks flat

c. The barrel-shaped chest is seen

d. Lung field lucency is increased

47. A pulmonary embolus is visible in the lungs of a dead person. Which of the following will prove that the embolus was formed before death?

a. Hypoxemia

b. Tachypnea

c. Lines of Zahn

d. Ghon's complex

48. Which is the imaging test of choice for pulmonary emboli?

a. Chest X-ray

b. CT pulmonary angiography

c. Pulse oximetry

d. Spirometry

49. The physician asks the nurse to assess the alveolar sputum sample. The nurse saw golden brown shaped bodies in the sample test. What is the diagnosis based on this finding?

a. Bronchiectasis

b. Asbestosis

c. Berylliosis

d. Silicosis

50. "Ivory white" calcified plaque deposits in the pleura and above the diaphragm are seen in:

a. Coal workers' pneumoconiosis

b. Asbestosis

c. Berylliosis

d. Silicosis

51. Which lung disease is also known as "black lung disease"?

a. Mesothelioma

b. Coal workers' pneumoconiosis

c. Atelectasis

d. Tension pneumothorax

52. When the asthmatic attack is seen more than two times a week but not daily, it is known as:

a. Intermittent asthma

b. Mild asthma

c. Moderate asthma

d. Severe asthma

53. A patient is suffering from asthma. He gave a history of alcohol consumption daily for 25 years. Which of the following drug should not be prescribed?

a. Albuterol

b. Zileuton

c. Montelukast

d. Ipratropium

54. An asthmatic patient is prescribed dextromethorphan. She was admitted with difficulty in breathing, unsteadiness, and hallucinations. Which of these drugs can be used to treat the patient?

a. Naloxone

b. Diphenhydramine

c. Iloprost

d. Cetirizine

55. Central chest pain can occur due to:

a. Massive pulmonary embolism

b. Bronchitis

c. Esophageal disease

d. Heart disease

56. Plexiform lesions are a characteristic feature of:

a. Pleural effusion

b. Pneumonia

c. Tuberculosis

d. Pulmonary hypertension

57. The physician asks the nurse to read the chest X-ray. The nurse observes hyperinflation and bullae in the CXR. What can be the diagnosis based on these findings?

a. Acute severe asthma

b. Pulmonary edema

c. Massive pulmonary embolus

d. Acute exacerbation of COPD pneumonia

58. A patient was admitted to the hospital with symptoms including fever, cough, shortness of breath, and loss of taste. Which of these is the most probable diagnosis?

a. Allergic rhinitis

b. Common cold

c. Covid-19

d. Influenza

59. Goodpasture disease can lead to (Select all that apply)

a. Dry cough

b. Dyspnea

c. Hemoptysis

d. Pulmonary hemorrhage

60. Which of these is the most common cause of mortality in Goodpasture disease?

a. Kidney failure

b. Pulmonary hemorrhage

c. Dyspnea

d. Edema

61. The lung biopsy report states hypertrophy of mucous secreting glands in the bronchioles. Which of the following is the most probable diagnosis?

a. Asthma

b. Chronic bronchitis

c. Pneumonia

d. Pulmonary embolism

62. Homan's sign is a characteristic feature of:

a. Deep vein thrombosis

b. Pulmonary embolism

c. Emphysema

d. Bronchiectasis

63. Which drug can be used as an antidote for acetaminophen overdose?

a. N-acetylcysteine

b. Dextromethorphan

c. Loratadine

d. Naloxone

64. Which of the following lung cancer is most common in non-smokers?

a. Squamous cell carcinoma

b. Large cell carcinoma

c. Adenocarcinoma

d. Small cell carcinoma

65. The drug of choice to treat lung abscess is:

a. Clindamycin

b. Azithromycin

c. Penicillin

d. Amoxicillin

66. Select the statements true for Acute respiratory distress syndrome. (Select all that apply).

a. Sudden dyspnea occurs in ARDs.

b. Capillary permeability is increased.

c. Oxygen therapy does not help in the treatment.

d. It is frequently associated with the dysfunction of other organs.

67. On the chest X-ray, "Eggshell" calcification is visible in hilar lymph nodes. What is the diagnosis based on this finding?

a. Asbestosis

b. Berylliosis

c. Silicosis

d. Black lung disease

68. Upper lobes of the lungs are usually not affected in:

a. Asbestosis

b. Berylliosis

c. Silicosis

d. Black lung disease

69. Which of the following statement is not true for idiopathic pulmonary fibrosis? (Select all that apply)

a. It is commonly seen between 40-50 years of age.

b. A nonproductive cough is a common symptom.

c. Fine inspiratory crackles are not heard on auscultation.

d. Digital clubbing is seen.

70. In the chest X-ray of bronchial carcinoma (Select all that apply)

a. Hilar mass is seen

b. Depression of hemidiaphragm is visible

c. Rib destruction can be seen

d. Pleural effusion is visible

71. Which of these is not a systemic presentation of extrapulmonary TB? (Select all that apply)

a. Cranial nerve palsy

b. Scoliosis

c. Abdominal mass

d. Transudative ascites

72. Which of these is not a correct drug for the treatment of severe community-acquired pneumonia?

a. Clarithromycin 500 mg IV twice daily + Co-amoxiclav 1.2 g

IV 3 times daily

b. Co-amoxiclav 1.2 g IV 3 times daily + erythromycin 500 mg–1 g IV 4 times daily

c. Ceftriaxone 1–2 g daily + Co-amoxiclav 1.2 g IV 3 times daily

d. Clarithromycin 500 mg IV twice daily + erythromycin 500 mg–1 g IV 4 times daily

73. The complications of pneumonia are: (Select all that apply)

a. Emphysema

b. Lobar collapse

c. Pneumothorax

d. Lung abscess

74. The clinical findings of bronchiectasis are:

a. Hemoptysis

b. Purulent sputum

c. Digital clubbing

d. Mucus plugging

75. Which of these is/are common complaint/complaints of vocal cord dysfunction? (Select all that apply)

a. Chronic cough

b. Dyspnea

c. Throat tightness

d. Nausea

76. While taking a sample for coronavirus disease, the swab should be entered: (Select all that apply)

a. Parallel to the floor of nostril

b. Till hindrance is felt when you reach posterior nasopharynx

c. Nasopharynx

d. And left for 2 minutes

77. Which of these causes pulmonary hypertension?

a. Heredity

b. Amphetamine

c. Fibrosis of lung

d. Congenital heart disease

78. The findings that indicate the progression of Covid-19 to pneumonia are: (Select all that apply)

a. Lymphocytopenia

b. Ground-glass opacities on CT scan

c. Thickening of Intralobular sputum

d. Elevated CRP

79. Common transmission modes of Covid-19 include: (Select all that apply)

a. Contaminated water

b. Direct contact

c. Fomites

d. Respiratory droplets

80. The suitable conditions to store the nasopharyngeal specimen taken to test Covid-19 are (Select all that apply):

a. The specimen can be stored at 15°C for 72 hours.

b. To store the specimen for a longer duration, the appropriate temperature is -70°C

c. The specimens cannot be stored for more than 72 hours.

d. The specimen can be stored at 2-8°C for 72 hours.

81. Permanently dilated airways are seen in bronchiectasis. (True/False)

82. If SpO_2
< 93% in a person with Covid-19, Oxygen therapy of 1-6L O_2/min is
recommended via cannula. (True/False)

83. The incubation period of SARS CoV-2 is 10-18 days. (True/False)

84. A negative tuberculin test result can be obtained if the BCG vaccine was administered in person. (True/False)

85. Gram and Ziehl-Neelsen stain is used for microscopy of sputum samples in the diagnosis of Tuberculosis. (True/False)

86. Chest physiotherapy is not needed in the management of cystic fibrosis. (True/False)

87. Sometimes, breathlessness is the only symptom in Bronchiectasis. (True/False)

88. Cyanosis is a common symptom in emphysema and chronic
bronchitis. (True/False)

89. Large pulmonary emboli can cause sudden death. (True/False)

90. Caplan syndrome is a combination of osteoarthritis and pneumoconiosis. (True/False)

91. Malignancy of
pleura along with asbestosis is known as Mesothelioma. (True/False)

92. PaO_2 is normal during the day in sleep apnea. (True/False)

93. Obesity hypoventilation syndrome is also called Pickwickian syndrome. (True/False)

94. Hyperresonant percussion is a finding of atelectasis on lung examination. (True/False)

95. Traumatic pneumothorax can be caused by gunshot. (True/False)

96. Bronchopneumonia is also known as walking pneumonia. (True/False)

97. Generally, the CXR in asthma shows opacities. (True/False)

98. A person suffering from emphysema is usually thin and barrel-chested. (True/False)

99. Superadded bacterial pneumonia is a common complication
of influenza. (True/False)

100. Chronic bronchitis is diagnosed by spirometry and methacholine test. (True/false)

101. Succinycholine is contraindicated in a client diagnosed with:

a. Asthma

b. Recent Stroke

c. Renal Failure

d. CHF

102. Assist control on a ventilator provides:

a. Sets the rate and tidal volume on the patient's initiative.

b. Spontaneous breaths are not supplemented.

c. Supports each spontaneous breath with supplemental flow to achieve a preset pressure.

d. None of the above

103. What could cause a high-pressure alarm on a patient's ventilator?

a. Kinked tube

b. Client biting on tube

c. Secretions in tube

d. All the above

104. Bronchial sounds heard in areas other than large airways may indicate?

a. Pneumonia

b. Pulmonary edema

c. COPD

d. Stridor

105. When caring for a patient with emphysema, the nurse assesses the oxygen flow rate to ensure that it does not exceed:

a. 2L/min

b. 6L/min

c. 4L/min

d. 10L/min

106. The purpose of pursed lip breathing is:

a. Promote carbon dioxide elimination

b. Strengthen the diaphragm

c. Strengthen the alveoli in the lungs

d. None of the above

107. When assessing for signs and symptoms of right sided heart failure, the nurse looks for:

a. Peripheral edema

b. Hypertension

c. clubbing of the nails

d. Increased appetite

108. The physician has scheduled a client for a left pneumonectomy. The position that will most likely be ordered postoperatively

is:

a. Prone

b. Nonoperative side or back

c. Either side is as long as patient is comfortable

d. Operative side or back

109. Which of the following organisms most commonly causes

community-acquired pneumonia in adults?

a. Streptococcus pneumoniae

b. Hemophilus influenzae

c. Staphylococcus aureus

d. Klebsiella pneumoniae

110. A client has active TB. Which of the following symptoms will he exhibit?

a. Headache and photophobia

b. Chills. fever. night sweats. and hemoptysis

c. Fever of more than 104*F and nausea

d. Lower back pain

Respiratory Nursing Review Questions With Answers and Rationales:

1. The first and most common symptom of emphysema is:

a. Purulent sputum

b. Episodic wheezing

c. Cough

d. Dyspnea

Answer: (d) Dyspnea is the most common and the first symptom of Emphysema. It begins gradually but shows a steady progression.

2. The physician suspects bronchiectasis in a patient. Which test will he ask the nurse to perform to confirm the diagnosis?

a. Lung biopsy

b. Chest CT scan

c. Blood test

d. Bronchoscopy

Answer: (b) Chest CT scan can give a clear image to confirm the diagnosis. The chest CT scan shows dilated, thickened airways that are commonly seen in the disease.

3. The "pink puffers" are the patients of disease:

a. Tuberculosis

b. Emphysema

c. Asthma

d. Pneumonia

Answer: (b) Emphysema is the disease in which the person suffers from shortness of breath and thus breaths fast. The skin appears pink in color. So, the patients are known as "pink puffers."

4. A patient comes to the physician and complains of symptoms like shortness of breath, wheezing, and tightness in the chest for a few months. What could be the diagnosis of his condition?

a. Pneumothorax

b. Tuberculosis

c. Asthma

d. Pneumonia

Answer: (c) Asthma is a condition in which the chronic inflammation and hyper-responsiveness of the airway lead to a triad of symptoms: shortness of breath, wheezing, and tightness.

5. A person suffering from asthma wants to get his wisdom tooth extracted. The dentist advised him to get a medical consent from his pulmonologist. What time will the pulmonologist advise him as the safest for getting the extraction done? (Select all that apply)

a. 9 AM

b. 11 AM

c. 2 PM

d. It is not safe at any time

Answer: (b) and (c) The safest time for an asthmatic patient to get the dental treatment done is late morning and early afternoon. The symptoms of asthma are worst early morning so, it should be avoided in the early morning time.

6. A person comes to the clinic and gives a history of his wife complaining about snoring and gasping sounds while sleeping. He also complains of sudden awakenings sometimes at night. Which of these is a probable cause of these symptoms?

a. Apnea

b. Tuberculosis

c. Sleep apnea

d. Cold

Answer: (d) Sleep apnea is a condition in which periodic cessation of breathing during sleeping leads to symptoms like snoring and gasping sounds. Sometimes, sudden awakenings occur while sleeping.

7. Which of the following is an obstructive pulmonary disease? (Select all that apply)

a. Chronic bronchitis

b. Pneumonia

c. Asthma

d. Emphysema

Answer: (a), (c), and (d) are obstructive pulmonary diseases because in all these diseases, blockage in the airway makes breathing difficult. Pneumonia is an inflammatory disease.

8. Using systemic corticosteroid in the treatment of severe asthma can lead to (Select all that apply)

a. Alteration of fat distribution

b. Glucose intolerance

c. Excitation of CNS

d. Delayed wound healing

e. Churg-Strauss syndrome

Answer: (a), (b) and (d) Using systemic corticosteroids in the treatment of asthma can give rise to cushingoid risks, alteration of fat distribution, glucose intolerance, delayed wound healing, and osteoporosis.

9. According to the modified MRC dyspnea scale, breathlessness after walking for a few minutes on level ground is considered as a grade:

a. 1

b. 2

c. 3

d. 4

Answer: (c) According to the modified MRC dyspnea scale, breathlessness after walking for a few minutes or 150 meters on level ground is considered as grade 3.

10. Select the key features of COPD. (Select all that apply)

a. Central cyanosis

b. Hyperinflated "barrel" chest

c. Non-palpable cardiac apex

d. Prolonged expiration

e. Use of accessory respiratory muscles

Answers: (a), (b), (c), (d) and (e)

In COPD, central cyanosis, symptoms like pursed-lip breathing, prolonged expiration, cardiac apex not palpable, hyperinflated "barrel" chest, use of accessory respiratory muscles, and auscultation are commonly seen.

11. Select the incorrect statement.

a. The functional residual cavity is residual volume + Expiratory reserve volume

b. Total lung capacity is inspiratory reserve volume + tidal volume + expiratory reserve volume

c. Inspiratory capacity is inspiratory reserve volume + tidal volume

d. Vital capacity is tidal volume + inspiratory reserve volume + expiratory reserve volume

Answer: (b)

Total lung capacity is inspiratory reserve volume + tidal volume + expiratory reserve volume + residual volume. It is the amount of air that can be accommodated in the lungs after a maximum inspiration. Its standard value is 6L.

12. The bronchus is not the primary obstructed site in:

a. Asthma

b. Emphysema

c. Chronic bronchitis

d. Bronchiectasis

Answer: (b) Emphysema is caused due to damage in the alveoli so, the primary obstructed site in emphysema is Alveoli.

13. An asthmatic patient informs the nurse that he is feeling gastric disturbances a few days after he started his treatment. Which of the following drug is most likely present in his regimen?

a. Beclometasone

b. Ipratropium

c. Theophylline

d. Montelukast

Answer: (c) Theophylline is the most potent bronchodilator. It has adverse effects on the GIT such as nausea, diarrhea, and vomiting.

14. Which of the following drugs are contraindicated in an asthmatic patient? (Select all that apply)

a. Ibuprofen

b. Losartan

c. Aspirin

d. Propranolol

Answer: (a), (c) and (d) Asthma can be precipitated by drugs like aspirin, NSAIDs (ibuprofen) and beta-blockers (propranolol). So, these are contraindicated in asthmatic patients.

15. A genetic respiratory disease caused by the mutation of a gene on chromosome 7 is:

a. Primary ciliary dyskinesia

b. Cystic fibrosis

c. Tracheoesophageal fistula

d. None of the above

Answer: (b) Cystic fibrosis is a genetic disorder seen due to mutation in the gene coding for transmembrane conductance regulator. Bronchiectasis is commonly seen in children suffering from this disorder.

16. A baby born prematurely during the 28th week of embryonic growth. Which of the following respiratory structure is most likely to be least developed?

a. Trachea

b. Bronchioles

c. Lungs

d. Alveoli

Answer: (d) The development of alveoli starts from 26th to 28th week of embryonic development. Development is seen in terms of the number and maturation of the alveoli after the 7th week of embryonic development. All other structures are developed until the 28th week.

17. A characteristic finding in the alveolus injured due to acute respiratory distress syndrome is:

a. Edema

b. Sloughed bronchial epithelium

c. Neutrophil sequestration and migration into alveolus

d. Hyaline membrane

Answer: (d) The Hyaline membrane is formed in the lining of the swollen alveolar ducts. This is a characteristic feature seen in the histological examination of alveolus injured due to acute respiratory distress syndrome.

18. While doing the lung examination, the nurse hears a fremitus sound. What can be the diagnosis based on this result?

a. Pneumothorax

b. Pleural effusion

c. Lobar pneumonia

d. Atelectasis

Answer: (c) In lobar pneumonia, fremitus lung sound is heard due to inflammation of the lung tissue. The lung tissue becomes denser.

19. A hypertensive patient came to the physician with a complaint of dry cough for 3 weeks. Which of these sentences are correct for this patient? (Select all that apply)

a. The patient is taking furosemide for hypertension.

b. The drug prescribed for hypertension needs to be replaced by alternative drug

c. The patient should be prescribed dextromethorphan for treating the dry cough permanently.

d. The patient is under captopril medication for hypertension.

Answer: (b) and (d)

Captopril is an ACE inhibitor used in the treatment of hypertension. The most common adverse effect of ACE inhibitors is a persistent dry cough. This cannot be treated permanently. The only treatment is the replacement of an ACE inhibitor with an alternative antihypertensive drug.

20. Pursed breathing is seen in: (Select all that apply)

a. Asthma

b. Chronic bronchitis

c. Emphysema

d. Bronchiectasis

Answer: (b) and (c) Pursed blip breathing is most commonly seen in chronic obstructive pulmonary diseases such as chronic bronchitis and emphysema.

21. Cervical or mediastinal lymphadenitis is commonly seen in:

a. Pulmonary tuberculosis

b. Miliary tuberculosis

c. Extrapulmonary tuberculosis

d. All the above

Answer: (c) Cervical lymphadenopathy is an enlargement of lymph nodes of the neck and mediastinal lymphadenopathy is an enlargement of mediastinal lymph nodes of the thorax. Cervical or mediastinal lymphadenitis is one of the most common presentations seen in extrapulmonary tuberculosis.

22. Clubbing of fingers is not seen due to:

a. Bronchiectasis

b. Lung abscess

c. Suppurative pneumonia

d. Massive pneumothorax

Answer: (d) Clubbing of fingers is seen due to increased soft tissue in the distal segments of fingers. This is seen due to lung disorders such as bronchiectasis, lung abscess, and suppurative pneumonia.

23. A nurse was assessing the chest wall movements in a patient. She observed bilateral diminished chest wall movements. What can be the diagnosis based on this finding?

a. Acute bronchitis

b. Bronchial asthma

c. Lobar collapse

d. Emphysema

Answer: (b) and (d) Chest wall movement is assessed by deep inspiration. Bilateral diminished chest wall movement is seen in diseases like bronchial asthma and emphysema. Chest wall movement is normal in acute bronchitis. In lobar collapse, chest wall movement is reduced on the affected side.

24. A type of asthma in which the patient does not get free from symptoms in between subsequent asthmatic attacks is:

a. Atopic asthma

b. Status asthmaticus

c. Chronic asthma

d. non-atopic asthma

Answer: (b) In status asthmaticus, the person does not get free from the symptoms of the previous attack before the onset of the next attack. The symptoms can remain throughout the day or night.

25. Which of the following is most commonly caused by aspiration of oropharyngeal contents?

a. Lung abscess

b. Lung cancer

c. Pneumonia

d. Pneumothorax

Answer: (a) Lung abscess is caused due to accumulation of the pus in the parenchyma cells of the lungs. It is commonly seen when oropharyngeal contents are aspirated.

26. A patient is prescribed theophylline. What should the common adverse effect be informed to the patient?

a. Diarrhea

b. Tremors

c. Tachycardia

d. Candidiasis

Answer: (a) Common adverse effects of theophylline include GI disturbances such as nausea, diarrhea, and vomiting. Other side effects are tachycardia and anxiety.

27. Which of the following is caused by rhinovirus?

a. Nasal polyp

b. Rhinitis

c. Bronchitis

d. Nasopharyngeal carcinoma

Answer: (b) Rhinitis is inflammation of the nasal mucosa that is caused by the rhinovirus. Its symptoms are runny nose, sneezing, and congestion.

28. Consolidation of an entire lobe of the lung visible in the chest X-ray of is a diagnostic feature of:

a. Lobar pneumonia

b. Bronchopneumonia

c. Aspiration pneumonia

d. Atypical pneumonia

Answer: (a) Lobar pneumonia is caused by a bacterial infection of streptococcus pneumonia. In this, the consolidation of an entire lobe is seen. Instead of air, the lobe is filled with fluid.

29. A patient comes with a complaint of fever, cough, and difficulty in breathing for 8 days. He gives the history of alcohol consumption to the nurse. Which of the following can be the diagnosis based on this information?

a. Lobar pneumonia

b. Bronchopneumonia

c. Aspiration pneumonia

d. Atypical pneumonia

Answer: (c) Aspiration pneumonia is caused due to aspiration of contents into the respiratory tract. Aspiration of alcohol in the lungs can lead to aspiration pneumonia.

30. Which of the following is not prescribed to treat a dry cough?

a. Dextromethorphan

b. Codeine

c. Bromhexine

d. Noscapine

Answer: (c) For dry (nonproductive cough), codeine, pholcodine, noscapine, and dextromethorphan are used. Bromhexine is used in the treatment of productive cough.

31. Which of these is not true for broncho-pneumonia?

a. Bronchial and bronchiolar inflammation is seen.

b. Consolidation is seen in an entire lobe.

c. More commonly seen in lower lobes.

d. None of these

Answer: (b) Consolidation in the entire lobe is seen in lobar pneumonia. In broncho-pneumonia, a patchy consolidation is seen in the alveolar region.

32. A patient was recently admitted to the hospital with the symptoms of shortness of breath, fever, and cough. After looking at his chest X-ray, pneumonia was diagnosed. The patient gave the history of international travel 1 month ago. Which of these can be the most probable diagnosis? (Select all that apply)

a. Acute respiratory distress syndrome

b. Coronavirus disease

c. Severe acute respiratory syndrome

d. Tuberculosis

Answer: (a) and (b) In 2019-2020, coronavirus pandemic occurred in the world. It was more commonly seen in people with a history of international travel or contact with a person with a history of international travel. Severe lung damage occurs in the disease that leads to acute respiratory distress syndrome. It is one of the causes of death in coronavirus disease.

33. An organism that causes pneumonia and is the third most common cause of urinary tract infection is:

a. Streptococcus pneumonia

b. Klebsiella pneumonia

c. Legionella

d. Burkholderia pseudomallei

Answer: (b) Klebsiella pneumoniae is a bacteria that causes pneumonia such as hospital-acquired pneumonia and aspiration pneumonia. It is the third most common cause of urinary tract infection.

34. The physician asks the nurse to perform the methacholine test. Which of the following diagnosis does the physician want to confirm?

a. Asthma

b. Pneumonia

c. Chronic bronchitis

d. Tuberculosis

Answer: (a) Methacholine test is used by administering an asthma triggering agent to check how the lung responds to the test. A drug is administered that causes the narrowing of the airway passages.

35. Microabsecess formation is a characteristic histologic feature of:

a. Community-acquired pneumonia

b. Suppurative pneumonia

c. Tuberculosis

d. Lobar pneumonia

Answer: (b) In suppurative pneumonia, pus accumulation occurs that results in the formation of micro abscesses formation. It can be seen in the chest X-ray as a dense opacity with cavity formation.

36. "Ghon focus" is a diagnostic feature of:

a. Pneumonia

b. Chronic bronchitis

c. Emphysema

d. Tuberculosis

Answer: (d) Tuberculosis is a bacterial disease caused by M. tuberculosis. "Ghon focus" is a mass of granuloma seen in the lung near the area of cessation. It is seen in tuberculosis.

37. A pregnant woman is diabetic. Which of these respiratory diseases may occur in the baby?

a. Respiratory distress syndrome

b. Pneumoniac. Acute bronchitis

d. Asthma

Answer: (a) When the mother is diabetic, neonatal respiratory distress syndrome may occur due to an increase in the concentration of fetal insulin. This affects the production of surfactant in the lungs of the baby.

38. Increased hemoglobin concentration is seen in:

a. Anemia

b. Polycythemiac. Leukemia

d. CO poisoning

Answer: (b) Polycythemia is a blood disorder in which the levels of hemoglobin are increased in the blood.

39. Trauma in the region of Kiesselbach plexus can lead to:

a. Rhinosinusitis

b. Epistaxisc. Deep vein thrombosis

d. Embolism

Answer: (b) Kiesselbach plexus is present in the anterior part of the nostril. Trauma at this plexus can lead to bleeding from the nose, known as epistaxis.

40. Which of the following drug can be added to the regimen if bronchodilator does not provide relief from asthma?

a. Inhaled steroid

b. High dose of steroidc. Corticosteroid and a sequential therapeutic drug

d. Oral steroid

Answer: (a) If bronchodilator does not provide relief from asthma, an inhaled steroid drug such as beclomethasone or sodium cromoglycate can be added to the regimen.

41. Lung abscess can be caused due to: (Select all that apply)

a. Pyogenic organisms

b. Thromboembolism of lungc. M. tuberculosis

d. Smoking

Answer: (a), (b) and (c) Lung abscess can be caused due to necrotizing infection by a pyogenic organism such as Staphylococcus aureus and klebsiella. It can be caused due to M. tuberculosis. Thromboembolism of lung can also lead to lung abscess.

42. Which of the following is not a cause of pleural effusion?

a. Increased production of the fluid

b. Reduced fluid absorption by pleura

c. Decreased capillary permeability

d. Increased hydrostatic pressure.

Answer: (c) When the capillary permeability is increased, leakage of the fluids from the capillaries in the pleural cavity occurs. This causes accumulation of the fluid and, thus, pleural effusion.

43. Which fluid is accumulated in chylothorax?

a. Blood

b. Pus

c. Chyme

d. Chyle

Answer: (c) Chyle is the milky fluid rich in triglycerides present in the lacteals of the small intestine. Due to the disruption in the thoracic duct, chyle gets accumulated in the pleural space. This causes chylothorax.

44. Select the incorrect statements for tuberculous pleural effusion. (Select all that apply)

a. Transudate fluid

b. Lymphocytes are predominant cells

c. The fluid is straw-colored

d. The fluid is blood-stained

Answer: (a) and (d) In tuberculous pleural effusion, a straw-colored exudate is accumulated in the pleural space. It is a common cause of extrapulmonary tuberculosis.

45. The pathologic report of bronchi states the presence of Charcot-Leyden crystals. What can be the diagnosis based on this finding?

a. Emphysema

b. Chronic bronchitis

c. Asthma

d. Pneumonia

Answer: (c) In asthma, eosinophilic needle-like crystals are seen as pathology in the bronchioles. These crystals are known as Charcot-Leyden crystals and are formed due to the breakdown of eosinophils in the sputum.

46. In the chest X-ray of a patient suffering from emphysema: (Select all that apply)

a. Anteroposterior diameter of the chest is increased

b. Diaphragm looks flat

c. The barrel-shaped chest is seen

d. Lung field lucency is increased

Answer: (a), (b), (c), and (d) In emphysema, enlargement of air spaces is seen. The findings on the chest X-ray are increased anteroposterior diameter of the chest, increased lung field latency, flattening of the diaphragm, and barrel-shaped chest.

47. A pulmonary embolus is visible in the lungs of a dead person. Which of the following will prove that the embolus was formed before death?

a. Hypoxemia

b. Tachypnea

c. Lines of Zahn

d) Ghon's complex

Answer: (c) Lines of Zahn are the pink and red areas seen in the embolus. These areas prove that the embolus was formed before death. Pink areas are due to platelets and fibrin. Red areas are due to RBCs.

48. Which is the imaging test of choice for pulmonary emboli?

a. Chest X-ray

b. CT pulmonary angiography

c. Pulse oximetry

d. Spirometry

Answer: (b) CT pulmonary angiography is a medical test done to obtain a CT scan image of the arteries of the lungs. This is done to check for embolism in the pulmonary arteries.

49. The physician asks the nurse to assess the alveolar sputum sample. The nurse saw golden brown and shaped bodies in the sample test. What is the diagnosis based on this finding?

a. Bronchiectasis

b. Asbestosis

c. Berylliosis

d. Silicosis

Answer: (b) Asbestosis is a respiratory pathology caused by inhalation of asbestoses particle. In the alveolar sputum sample, golden-brown shaped asbestoses bodies are present. These can be seen when stained by Prussian blue stain.

50. "Ivory white" calcified plaque deposits in the pleura and above the diaphragm are seen in:

a. Coal workers' pneumoconiosis

b. Asbestosis

c. Berylliosis

d. Silicosis

Answer: (b) In asbestoses, "ivory white" calcified deposits are seen above the diaphragm and in the pleura.

51. Which lung disease is also known as "black lung disease"?

a. Mesothelioma

b. Coal workers' pneumoconiosis

c. Atelectasis

d. Tension pneumothorax

Answer: (b) Black lung disease or coal worker pneumoconiosis is a lung disorder caused by long term inhalation of the coal particles. It is commonly seen in coal miners and other people that work in the coal industry.

52. When the asthmatic attack is seen more than two times a week but not daily, it is known as:

a. Intermittent asthma

b. Mild asthma

c. Moderate asthma

d. Severe asthma

Answer: (b) When the asthmatic attack is seen less than two times a day, it is considered intermittent. When it is seen more than twice a week, it is considered mild. When it occurs daily, it is considered moderate. In severe asthma, the symptoms are seen daily and are very extreme. It can sometimes occur twice a day.

53. A patient is suffering from asthma. He gave a history of alcohol consumption daily for 25 years. Which of the following drug should not be prescribed?

a. Albuterol

b. Zileuton

c. Montelukast

d. Ipratropium

Answer: (b) Zileuton is an anti-leukotriene drug used in the treatment of asthma. It can lead to hepatotoxicity. The liver is already weak in people drinking alcohol for a long time so, this drug should not be prescribed in such patients.

54. An asthmatic patient is prescribed dextromethorphan. She was admitted with difficulty in breathing, unsteadiness, and hallucinations. Which of these drugs can be used to treat the patient?

a. Naloxone

b. Diphenhydramine

c. Iloprost

d. Cetirizine

Answer: (a) Dextromethorphan is an opioid drug. Its overdose is harmful and can lead to an increased heartbeat, difficulty in breathing, unsteadiness, and hallucinations. This can be treated by an antidotal therapy using Naloxone as it is an opioid antagonist.

55. Central chest pain can occur due to:

a. Massive pulmonary embolism

b. Bronchitis

c. Esophageal disease

d. Heart disease

Answer: (b) In bronchitis, chest discomfort is seen. Central chest pain is usually not seen.

56. Plexiform lesions are a characteristic feature of:

a. Pleural effusion

b. Pneumonia

c. Tuberculosis

d. Pulmonary hypertension

Answer: (d) In pulmonary hypertension, hypertrophy of the vessel wall occurs. Hypertrophy occurs in the epithelial cells. These changes appear as plexiform lesions.

57. The physician asks the nurse to read the chest X-ray. The nurse observes hyperinflation and bullae in the CXR. What can be the diagnosis based on these findings?

a. Acute severe asthma

b. Pulmonary edema

c. Massive pulmonary embolus

d. Acute exacerbation of COPD pneumonia

Answer: (d) In acute exacerbation of COPD pneumonia, the findings are seen on the CXR are hyperinflation, bullae, and pneumonic consolidation. Hyperinflation is also seen in severe acute asthma, but bullae are usually not present.

58. A patient was admitted to the hospital with symptoms including fever, cough, shortness of breath, and loss of taste. Which of these is the most probable diagnosis?

a. Allergic rhinitis

b. Common cold

c. Covid-19

d. Influenza

Answer: (c) Covid-19 is a disease that leads to a pandemic in 2019-2020. The common symptoms of the disease are fever, cough, shortness of breath, fatigue, and loss of taste.

59. Goodpasture disease can lead to (Select all that apply)

a. Dry cough

b. Dyspnea

c. Hemoptysis

d. Pulmonary hemorrhage

Answer: (a), (b), (c) and (d) Goodpasture disease affects the kidney and lungs. Common respiratory symptoms are dry cough, dyspnea, hemoptysis, and pulmonary hemorrhage.

60. Which of these is the most common cause of mortality in Goodpasture disease?

a. Kidney failure

b. Pulmonary hemorrhage

c. Dyspnea

d. Edema

Answer: (b) Massive pulmonary hemorrhage is a characteristic feature of Goodpasture disease. It is the most common cause of death due to this disease.

61. The lung biopsy report states hypertrophy of mucous secreting glands in the bronchioles. Which of the following is the most probable diagnosis?

a. Asthma

b. Chronic bronchitis

c. Pneumonia

d. Pulmonary embolism

Answer: (b) In chronic bronchitis, hypertrophy and hyperplasia of the mucous secreting glands are seen in the bronchioles. It is visible in the biopsy report.

62. Homan's sign is a characteristic feature of:

a. Deep vein thrombosis

b. Pulmonary embolism

c. Emphysema

d. Bronchiectasis

Answer: (a) Homan's sign is seen in deep vein thrombosis where the calf muscle feels tender during dorsiflexion of the foot.

63. Which drug can be used as an antidote for acetaminophen overdose?

a. N-acetylcysteine

b. Dextromethorphan

c. Loratadine

d. Naloxone

Answer: (a) N-acetylcysteine is a mucolytic drug used in the treatment of COPD. It is also in acetaminophen overdose as an antidote.

64. Which of the following lung cancer is most common in non-smokers?

a. Squamous cell carcinoma

b. Large cell carcinoma

c. Adenocarcinoma

d. Small cell carcinoma

Answer: (c) The most common lung cancer in nonsmokers is adenocarcinoma. The glandular pattern is seen in the histology of the tissue.

65. The drug of choice to treat lung abscess is:

a. Clindamycin

b. Azithromycin

c. Penicillin

d. Amoxicillin

Answer: (a) For the treatment of lung abscess, a broad-spectrum antibiotic is preferred. Clindamycin is the preferred antibiotic.

66. Select the statements true for Acute respiratory distress syndrome. (Select all that apply).

a. Sudden dyspnea occurs in ARDs.

b. Capillary permeability is increased.

c. Oxygen therapy does not help in the treatment.

d. It is frequently associated with the dysfunction of other organs.

Answer: (a), (b), and (d) In ARDS, sudden breathlessness is common. Other characteristics features are increased capillary permeability and pulmonary edema. Oxygen therapy is used to ensure an adequate flow of oxygen. It is associated with dysfunction of other organs that can lead to multiorgan failure.

67. On the chest X-ray, "Eggshell" calcification is visible in hilar lymph nodes. What is the diagnosis based on this finding?

a. Asbestosis

b. Berylliosis

c. Silicosis

d. Black lung disease

Answer: (c) In silicosis, "eggshell" calcification is seen on the chest X-ray due to the inhalation of silica particles.

68. Upper lobes of the lungs are usually not affected in:

a. Asbestosis

b. Berylliosis

c. Silicosis

d. Black lung disease

Answer: (a) In asbestosis, lower lobes of the lung are affected.

69. Which of the following statement is not true for idiopathic pulmonary fibrosis? (Select all that apply)

a. It is commonly seen between 40-50 years of age.

b. A nonproductive cough is a common symptom.

c. Fine inspiratory crackles are not heard on auscultation.

d. Digital clubbing is seen.

Answer: (a) and (c) Idiopathic pulmonary fibrosis is usually not seen before 50 years of age. Fine inspiratory crackles similar to the sound while parting the Velcro is heard on auscultation.

70. In the chest X-ray of bronchial carcinoma (Select all that apply)

a. Hilar mass is seen

b. Depression of hemidiaphragm is visible

c. Rib destruction can be seen

d. Pleural effusion is visible

Answer: (a), (c), and (d) Common radiologic features of bronchial carcinoma are hilar mass, the elevation of hemidiaphragm, rib destruction, pleural effusion, and peripheral opacity.

71. Which of these is not a systemic presentation of extrapulmonary TB? (Select all that apply)

a. Cranial nerve palsy

b. Scoliosis

c. Abdominal mass

d. Transudative ascites

Answer: (b) and (d) systemic presentation of extrapulmonary TB include kyphosis and exudative ascites formation.

72. Which of these is not a correct drug for the treatment of severe community-acquired pneumonia?

a. Clarithromycin 500 mg IV twice daily + Co-amoxiclav 1.2 g IV 3 times daily

b. Co-amoxiclav 1.2 g IV 3 times daily + erythromycin 500 mg–1 g IV 4 times daily

c. Ceftriaxone 1–2 g daily + Co-amoxiclav 1.2 g IV 3 times daily

d. Clarithromycin 500 mg IV twice daily + erythromycin 500 mg–1 g IV 4 times daily

Answer: (c) and (d) For the treatment of severe community-acquired pneumonia, Clarithromycin 500 mg IV twice daily or erythromycin 500 mg–1 g IV 4 times daily should be used along with Co-amoxiclav 1.2 g IV 3 times daily or ceftriaxone 1–2 g daily or cefuroxime 1.5 g 3 times daily.

73. The complications of pneumonia are: (Select all that apply)

a. Emphysema

b. Lobar collapse

c. Pneumothorax

d. Lung abscess

Answer: (a), (b), (c), and (d) Common complications of pneumonia are emphysema, parapneumonic effusion, lobar collapse, lung abscess, pneumothorax, and thromboembolic disease.

74. The clinical findings of bronchiectasis are:

a. Hemoptysis

b. Purulent sputum

c. Digital clubbing

d. Mucus plugging

Answer: (a), (b), and (c) In bronchiectasis, mucus plugging is not seen. Characteristic clinical findings are hemoptysis, purulent sputum, digital clubbing, and recurrent infections.

75. Which of these is/are common complaint/complaints of vocal cord dysfunction? (Select all that apply)

a. Chronic cough

b. Dyspnea

c. Throat tightness

d. Nausea

Answer: (a), (b) and (c) In vocal cord dysfunction, the most common clinical symptoms are chronic cough, hoarseness, dyspnea, tightness in the throat, aphonia, and dysphonia.

76. While taking a sample for coronavirus disease, the swab should be entered: (Select all that apply)

a. Parallel to the floor of nostril

b. Till hindrance is felt when you reach posterior nasopharynx

c. Nasopharynx

d. And left for 2 minutes

Answer: (a), (b), and (c) To collect the nasopharyngeal specimen, a synthetic fiber swab attached to a small plastic shaft should be entered straight in the nostril. It should be inserted parallel to the floor of the nostril. It should be entered until it reaches the posterior nasopharynx. It is left for a few seconds to absorb the contents in the swab.

77. Which of these causes pulmonary hypertension?

a. Heredity

b. Amphetamine

c. Fibrosis of lung

d. Congenital heart disease

Answer: (a), (b) and (d) Pulmonary hypertension can be idiopathic or hereditary. Drugs like amphetamine and codeine can cause it too. It is also caused due to congenital heart disease, HIV, and portal hypertension.

78. The findings that indicate the progression of Covid-19 to pneumonia are: (Select all that apply)

a. Lymphocytopenia

b. Ground-glass opacities on CT scan

c. Thickening of Intralobular sputum

d. Elevated CRP

Answer: (a), (b), (c) and (d) Severity of Covid-19 disease increases when it progresses to pneumonia. The findings that indicate the progression are lymphocytopenia, ground glass appearance on CT scan, elevated CRP and thickening of the intralobular sputum.

79. Common transmission modes of Covid-19 include: (Select all that apply)

a. Contaminated water

b. Direct contact

c. Fomites

d. Respiratory droplets

Answer: (b), (c), and (d) Covid-19 transmission occur by respiratory droplets of an infected person and direct contact with the infected person. Fomites or surfaces made of aluminum, glass, or stainless steel also transmit the disease. Contaminated water due to feces of an infected person can transmit the disease too, but the chances are low.

80. The suitable conditions to store the nasopharyngeal specimen taken to test Covid-19 are:

a. The specimen can be stored at 15°C for 72 hours.

b. To store the specimen for a longer duration, the appropriate temperature is -70°C

c. The specimens cannot be stored for more than 72 hours.

d. The specimen can be stored at 2-8°C for 72 hours.

Answer: (b),(d) Immediately after collecting the sample, it should be stored at 2-8°C when storage is needed only for 72 hours. If storage for longer duration is needed due to delayed transport or testing, it should be stored at -70°C.

81. Permanently dilated airways are seen in bronchiectasis. (True/False)

Answer: The statement is true. In bronchiectasis, chronic necrotizing infection in the bronchi results in permanent dilation of bronchi.

82. If SpO_2 < 93% in a person with Covid-19, Oxygen therapy of 1-6L O_2/min is recommended via cannula. (True/False)

Answer: The statement is true. Oxygen therapy is necessary when the SpO_2 is less than or equal to 93%. 1-6L O_2/min should be administered via nasal cannula.

83. The incubation period of SARS CoV-2 is 10-18 days. (True/False)

Answer: The statement is false. The incubation period of SARS CoV-2 is 2-14 days.

84. A negative tuberculin test result can be obtained if the BCG vaccine was administered in person. (True/False)

Answer: The statement is true. Tuberculin test results are negative when the person is exposed to the BCG vaccine or other non-tuberculous mycobacteria.

85. Gram and Ziehl-Neelsen stain is used for microscopy of sputum samples in the diagnosis of Tuberculosis. (True/False)

Answer: The statement is true. Mycobacterium is an acid-fast microorganism so, Ziehl-Neelsen stain is used along with Gram stain in the microbiology of sputum to diagnose tuberculosis.

86. Chest physiotherapy is not needed in the management of cystic fibrosis. (True/False)

Answer: The statement is false. Regular chest physiotherapy is helpful in the management of cystic fibrosis to improve airway clearance.

87. Sometimes, breathlessness is the only symptom in Bronchiectasis. (True/False)

Answer: The statement is false. Common symptoms of bronchiectasis are purulent sputum and hemoptysis. The disease in which breathlessness is the only symptom sometimes is pleural effusion.

88. Cyanosis is a common symptom in emphysema and chronic bronchitis. (True/False)

Answer: The statement is false. Cyanosis is a common symptom in chronic bronchitis due to reduced blood oxygen levels. It is not seen in emphysema as patients hyperventilate and are known as pink puffers.

89. Large pulmonary emboli can cause sudden death. (True/False)

Answer: The statement is true. A large pulmonary embolus reduces oxygen levels in the blood and affects the functions of the lung and other body tissues. This can lead to sudden death.

90. Caplan syndrome is a combination of osteoarthritis and pneumoconiosis. (True/False)

Answer: The statement is false. Caplan syndrome is a combination of rheumatoid arthritis and pneumoconiosis. It is also called as rheumatoid pneumoconiosis.

91. Malignancy of pleura along with asbestosis is known as Mesothelioma. (True/False)

Answer: The statement is true. Mesothelioma is a tumor seen in the lining of the lungs, heart, and abdomen. It is caused by asbestos fibers.

92. PaO_2 is normal during the day in sleep apnea. (True/False)

Answer: The statement is true. In sleep apnea, the PaO_2 is reduced during the night. It remains normal during the daytime.

93. Obesity hypoventilation syndrome is also called Pickwickian syndrome. (True/False)

Answer: The statement is true. In obesity hypoventilation syndrome, overweight or obese people suffer from hypoventilation due to difficulty in breathing. It is commonly called as Pickwickian syndrome.

94. Hyperresonant percussion is a finding of atelectasis on lung examination. (True/False)

Answer: The statement is false. A dull percussion sound is heard on lung examination in case of atelectasis.

95. Traumatic pneumothorax can be caused by gunshot. (True/False)

Answer: The statement is true. A penetrating gunshot can damage the airway or lung tissues. This can result in the accumulation of air in the pleural space.

96. Bronchopneumonia is also known as walking pneumonia. (True/False)

Answer: The statement is false. Walking pneumonia is atypical or interstitial pneumonia. It is less severe pneumonia.

97. Generally, the CXR in asthma shows opacities. (True/False)

Answer: The statement is false. The CXR is generally normal in most of the asthmatic patients.

98. A person suffering from emphysema is usually thin and barrel-chested. (True/False)

Answer: The statement is true. In emphysema, the person loses weight and is thin. The barrel-shaped chest is a common finding in emphysema.

99. Superadded bacterial pneumonia is a common complication of influenza. (True/False)

Answer: The statement is true. In influenza, the respiratory system is affected. Superadded bacterial or viral pneumonia is a common complication of the disease.

100. Chronic bronchitis is diagnosed by spirometry and methacholine test. (True/false)

Answer: The statement is false. Spirometry and methacholine test are used in the diagnosis of asthma.

101. Succinycholine is contraindicated in a client diagnosed with:

a. Asthma

b. Recent Stroke

c. Renal Failure

d. CHF

Answer: (C) Succinycholine is contraindicated in patients with Renal Failure.

102. Assist control on a ventilator provides:

a. Sets the rate and tidal volume on the patient's initiative.

b. Spontaneous breaths are not supplemented.

c. Supports each spontaneous breath with supplemental flow to achieve a preset pressure.

d. None of the above

Answer: (c) Assist control supports each spontaneous breath with supplemental flow to achieve a preset pressure.

103. What could cause a high-pressure alarm on a patient's ventilator?

a. Kinked tube

b. Client biting on tube

c. Secretions in tube

d. All the above

Answer: (d) All of these issues will cause high pressure in the tubing and cause a high-pressure alarm.

104. Bronchial sounds heard in areas other than large airways may indicate?

a. Pneumonia

b. Pulmonary edema

c. COPD

d. Stridor

Answer: (a) Bronchial sounds are usually indicative of pneumonia.

105. When caring for a patient with emphysema, the nurse assesses the oxygen flow rate to ensure that it does not exceed:

a. 2L/min

b. 6L/min

c. 4L/min

d. 10L/min

Answer: (a) 2L/min. Using oxygen therapy in patients with emphysema can be dangerous if not monitored carefully.

106. The purpose of pursed lip breathing is:

a. Promote carbon dioxide elimination

b. Strengthen the diaphragm

c. Strengthen the alveoli in the lungs

d. None of the above

Answer: (a) pursed lip breathing promotes carbon dioxide elimination. It provides a quick and easy way to slow your pace of breathing, making each breath more effective.

107. When assessing for signs and symptoms of right sided heart failure, the nurse looks for:

a. Peripheral edema

b. Hypertension

c. clubbing of the nails

d. Increased appetite

Answer: (a) Peripheral edema is one of the signs and symptoms of right sided heart failure. Shortness of breath, wheezing, fatigue, and dizziness are also signs of right sided heart failure.

108. The physician has scheduled a client for a left pneu-monectomy. The position that will most likely be ordered post-operatively is:

a. Prone

b. Nonoperative side or back

c. Either side is as long as patient is comfortable

d. Operative side or back

Answer: (d) Operative side or back is the best position for a pneumonectomy patient.

109. Which of the following organisms most commonly caus-es community-acquired pneumonia in adults?

a. Streptococcus pneumoniae

b. Hemophilus influenzae

c. Staphylococcus aureus

d. Klebsiella pneumoniae

Answer: (a) Streptococcus pneumoniae commonly causes community-acquired pneumonia in adults.

110. A client has active TB. Which of the following symptoms will he exhibit?

a. Headache and photophobia

b. Chills. fever. night sweats. and hemoptysis

c. Fever of more than 104*F and nausea

d. Lower back pain

Answer: (b) Chills. fever. night sweats. and hemoptysis are common signs of an active TB infection.